CONGRESS OF THE UNITED STATES
CONGRESSIONAL BUDGET OFFICE

A
CBO
PAPER

JANUARY 2007

Prescription Drug Pricing in the Private Sector

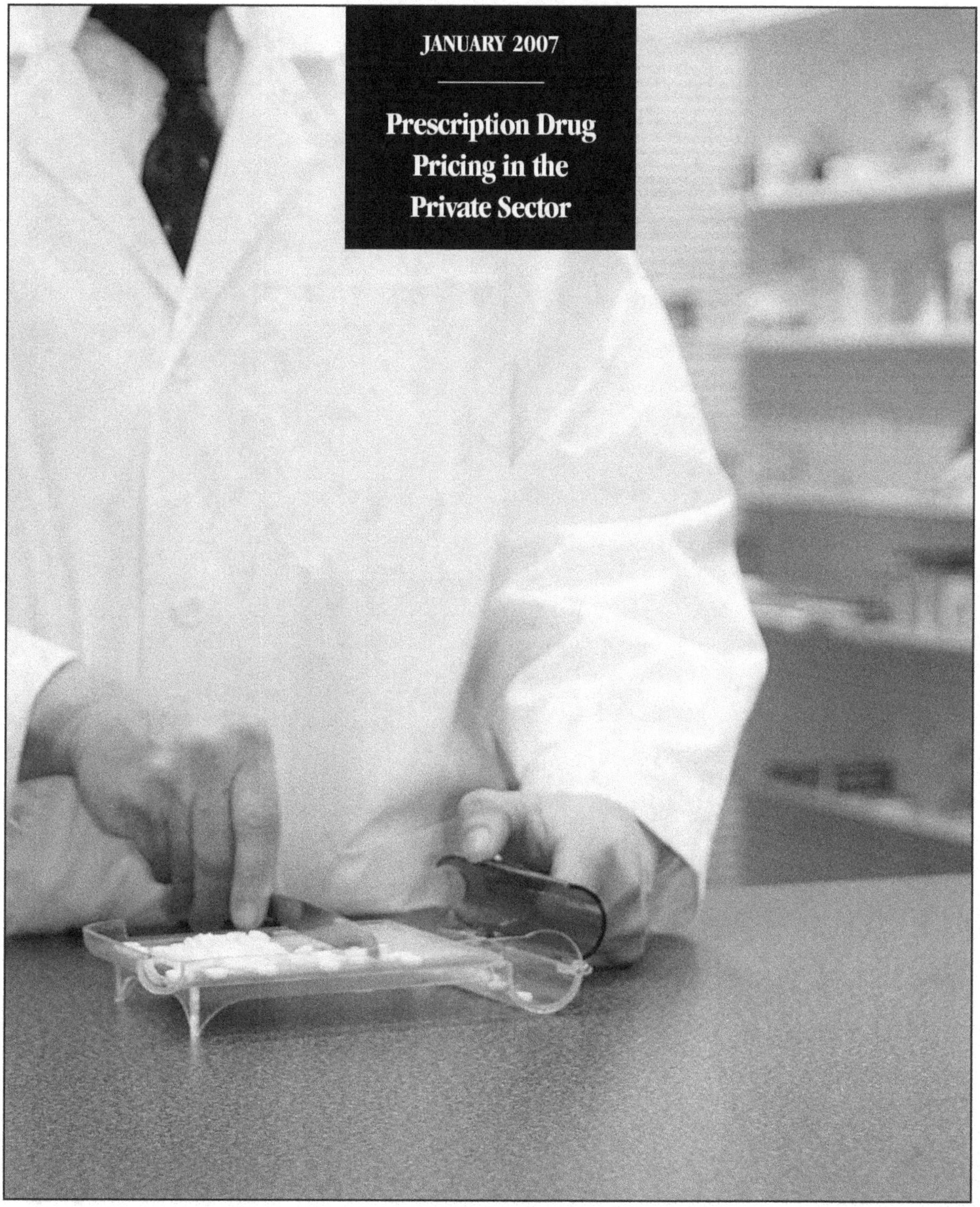

Pub. No. 2703

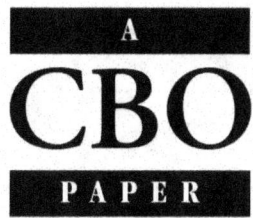

Prescription Drug Pricing in the Private Sector

January 2007

The Congress of the United States ■ Congressional Budget Office

Note

The numbers in the text, tables, and figures of this paper may not add up to totals because of rounding.

Preface

As prescription drugs move from manufacturers to consumers, a complex set of market transactions involving prices, discounts, and rebates occurs along the supply chain. Although the drugs themselves move in a relatively straightforward way, the flow of payments and the process by which they are determined are much more complex.

This Congressional Budget Office (CBO) paper, prepared at the request of Senate Majority Leader Frist, explains the supply chain, the flow of payments, and the process by which payments are determined and provides estimates of the relative prices that retail pharmacies and nonretail providers pay for prescription drugs. In keeping with CBO's mandate to provide objective, nonpartisan analysis, this paper makes no recommendations.

Julie Somers and Anna Cook prepared the paper under the supervision of Joseph Kile, David Moore, Bruce Vavrichek, and James Baumgardner. Alshadye Yemane and Susan Labovich assisted with the data analysis, and Peter Richmond assisted with the figures. Allison Percy served as CBO's internal reviewer. Information and data were provided by the Centers for Medicare & Medicaid Services as well as by IMS Health. Tom Bradley, Philip Ellis, Arlene Holen, Amy Petz, Shinobu Suzuki, and Tom Woodward provided useful comments on drafts. Outside of CBO, Terry Latanich and Judy Wagner, both private consultants, did the same. (The assistance of external reviewers implies no responsibility for the final product, which rests solely with CBO.)

John Skeen edited the paper, and Kate Kelly proofread it. Maureen Costantino took the photograph for the cover and prepared the paper for publication. Lenny Skutnik produced the printed copies, and Linda Schimmel handled the distribution.

Donald B. Marron
Acting Director

January 2007

Contents

Tables (Continued)

Figures

Boxes

Prescription Drug Pricing in the Private Sector

Summary

As prescription drugs move from manufacturers to consumers, a complex set of market transactions involving prices, discounts, and rebates occurs along the supply chain. Although the drugs themselves move in a relatively straightforward way from manufacturers to wholesalers to retail pharmacies or nonretail providers (such as hospitals and clinics) to final consumers, the flow of payments that occurs is more complicated. This Congressional Budget Office (CBO) paper explains the supply chain, the flow of payments, and the process by which payments are determined and provides estimates of the relative prices that retail pharmacies and nonretail providers pay for prescription drugs. Limitations in the available data preclude quantitative estimates of what consumers and health plans ultimately pay for prescription drugs, but this paper describes those participants' bargaining positions.

The prices that purchasers pay depend upon the degree of competition in a marketplace and on purchasers' bargaining power. In the pharmaceutical marketplace, competition depends on whether a brand-name drug has patent protection or whether brand-name and generic versions of the drug are both available. In addition, even brand-name drugs under patent protection can face competition from other brand-name drugs that are considered to be therapeutic substitutes.

A purchaser's bargaining power depends on both the volume purchased and the purchaser's ability to choose which drug to purchase from a set of competing drugs. For example, for brand-name drugs under patent protection, chain pharmacies and health plans may have different levels of success in negotiating lower prices from manufacturers even though they both may purchase a large volume of drugs. A chain pharmacy usually dispenses prescriptions as written by the physician for brand-name drugs under patent protection; so even though a chain pharmacy may buy a large volume of

brand-name drugs under patent protection, it generally cannot negotiate prices for them that are low compared with the prices negotiated by purchasers with more choice. In contrast, a health plan can choose to cover only one or two brand-name drugs from a set of drugs that are considered to be therapeutic substitutes; therefore, a health plan can negotiate lower prices from manufacturers (in the form of rebates) by buying a large volume of the brand-name drugs of the plan's choice.

In contrast, for generic drugs, the chain pharmacy, rather than the health plan, has greater negotiating leverage. The chain pharmacy can choose which of several generic drugs to stock, and it purchases large volumes of those drugs. Therefore, the chain pharmacy can negotiate lower prices from manufacturers for generic drugs. The health plan does not choose which generic drugs to dispense. Instead, the health plan's beneficiaries go to their pharmacies to fill prescriptions, and the pharmacies dispense the generic drugs that they have chosen to stock. Therefore, manufacturers have no incentive to negotiate price terms with a health plan for generic drugs even if the health plan buys a large volume of them.

The Supply Chain

Consumers obtain about three-quarters of their prescription drugs from retail pharmacies and the remainder from nonretail providers. Retail pharmacies include conventional outlets—chain pharmacies, independent pharmacies, and food stores with pharmacies—as well as the operationally different category of mail-order pharmacies (see Figure 1). Nonretail providers include hospitals, health maintenance organizations (HMOs), clinics, home health care providers, nursing homes, and federal facilities. The majority of drugs purchased by retail pharmacies and nonretail providers are purchased through wholesalers. Purchasing drugs from the pharmaceutical manufacturers, wholesalers decrease the number of transactions that would otherwise occur if the many retail

Figure 1.

The Supply Chain Through Which Drugs Are Delivered to Consumers

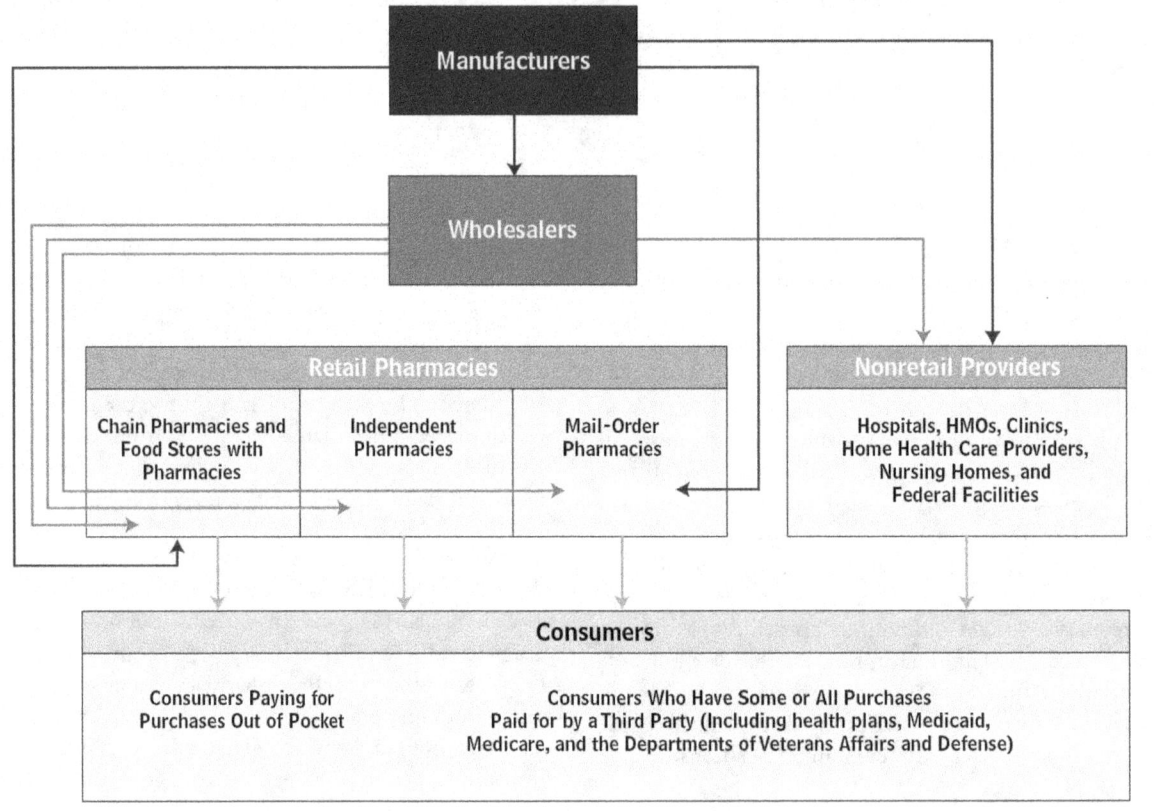

Source: Congressional Budget Office.

Note: HMO = health maintenance organization.

pharmacies and nonretail providers independently ordered from hundreds of manufacturers. Direct sales of drugs from manufacturers to retail pharmacies or non-retail providers generally involve purchasers large enough to internalize the wholesale function, like large chain pharmacies and food stores with pharmacies. Neverthe-less, even large chain pharmacies and food stores with pharmacies purchase a substantial portion of their drugs from wholesalers.

Retail pharmacies and nonretail providers negotiate drug prices with wholesalers or pharmaceutical manufacturers. In the retail pharmacy market, there are two additional negotiations: one between health plans or self-insured employers and the manufacturers and the other between health plans or self-insured employers and the retail phar-

macies. The health plans or self-insured employers often contract out those two additional negotiations to phar-macy benefit managers (PBMs). PBMs that organize a large number of patients under a formulary (a list of pre-ferred drugs) obtain discounted prices on many brand-name drugs in the form of rebates from manufacturers, which are in turn shared with health plans or self-insured employers. In 2004, nearly half of drug spending in the retail pharmacy market was covered by private health plans.[1]

---

1. See Centers for Medicare & Medicaid Services, National Health Expenditures by Type of Service and Source of Funds, 1960 to 2004, available at www.cms.hhs.gov/ NationalHealthExpendData/02_NationalHealthAccounts Historical.asp#TopOfPage.

Price Measures

There are three price measures that are important in understanding the payment system for prescription drugs in the retail pharmacy market: the average manufacturer price (AMP), the wholesale acquisition cost (WAC), and the average wholesale price (AWP). The AMP is an average of actual transaction prices. In contrast, the WAC and the AWP are list prices, like a sticker price in the automobile industry.

The AMP is the average price paid by wholesalers to manufacturers or by retail pharmacies that buy directly from manufacturers for drugs distributed through retail pharmacies. It reflects all rebates paid by manufacturers to wholesalers and to retail pharmacies. It does not include rebates paid by manufacturers to PBMs, Medicaid, or to other third-party payers. Manufacturers are required to report the AMP to the Department of Health and Human Services' Centers for Medicare & Medicaid Services (CMS), which uses it to calculate the rebates that manufacturers are required to pay state Medicaid programs for sales to Medicaid beneficiaries. For manufacturers, such rebates are a cost of participating in the Medicaid market.

The WAC represents manufacturers' published catalog, or list, price for sales of a drug (brand-name or generic) to wholesalers. However, in practice, the WAC is not what wholesalers pay for drugs. To the extent that the WAC is meaningful in conveying information about actual transaction costs, the utility is limited to single-source drugs (that is, brand-name drugs still under patent protection). For those drugs, the WAC often approximates the prices that retail pharmacies pay to wholesalers.

The AWP is a published list price for a drug sold by wholesalers to retail pharmacies and nonretail providers. However, in practice, the AWP is not what retail pharmacies and nonretail providers pay for drugs but, instead, is often used as a basis for payment to retail pharmacies by, for example, the Medicaid program, PBMs, and health plans. Those organizations often pay pharmacies a price discounted off of the AWP.

Single-Source Brand-Name Drugs

Using a sample of single-source prescription drugs in oral solid forms (that is, tablets and capsules) that accounted for over 40 percent of all U.S. drug sales in 2003, CBO analyzed the average prices that retail pharmacies and nonretail providers paid. Those price data—which CBO

purchased from IMS Health—do not reflect all of the discounts given by pharmaceutical manufacturers and so must be interpreted with caution. In particular, rebate payments from manufacturers are not captured in those prices.

Other prices analyzed in this paper do reflect rebate payments, but those prices cannot be attributed to a particular type of purchaser. An example is the "best price" reported to CMS under the Medicaid program. Manufacturers that choose to participate in the program must report the lowest price that any private-sector purchaser paid for a drug, including all discounts and rebates. Although CBO has analyzed those reported best prices, the purchasers who receive them are unknown.

According to CBO's analysis of the estimated average prices in the data from IMS Health, conventional retail pharmacies pay more for single-source brand-name drugs than do mail-order pharmacies and nonretail providers. That finding is not surprising because conventional pharmacies generally do not promote substitution among those drugs.[2] Rather, it is the other types of purchasers (mail-order pharmacies working on behalf of PBMs or health plans, and nonretail providers) who receive discounts by encouraging the substitution of one single-source brand-name drug for another.[3]

Mail-order pharmacies pay less for single-source brand-name drugs than do other retail pharmacies. When working on behalf of PBMs or health plans, mail-order pharmacies may have a greater ability to affect drugs' market shares for a large number of consumers—particularly for drugs that treat chronic conditions—compared with conventional pharmacies. The physician's permission is needed to switch from a more expensive brand-name drug to a therapeutically similar but less expensive drug. In a mail-order setting, pharmacists have additional time to contact physicians and attempt to obtain the needed permission. And because most of the prescriptions filled by mail-order pharmacies are for drugs that

2. When a pharmacy does contact a doctor to switch a prescription, it may be on behalf of a PBM or health plan using a formulary to manage the drug spending by its patients. The rebate would then go to the PBM or health plan, rather than to the pharmacy.

3. However, because limitations of the data kept CBO from estimating how much final purchasers paid retail pharmacies and nonretail providers, the agency also could not calculate the net amount that pharmacies and nonretail providers retained.

Table 1.

Average Prices for Single-Source Brand-Name Drugs Relative to the Average Wholesale Price

	Are Rebates That Are Not Reflected in the Price Shown Likely?	Average Price as a Percentage of AWP
Conventional Retail Pharmacies[a]	No	83
Mail-Order Pharmacies[b]	Yes	No More Than 78
Federal Facilities	No	42[c]
Nonretail Providers, Excluding Federal Facilities[d]	Yes	No More Than 74
Best Price	No	64

Source: Congressional Budget Office (CBO) based on data from IMS Health for the fourth quarter of 2003.

Notes: AWP = average wholesale price.

Mail-order pharmacies and nonretail providers can receive rebates from manufacturers on the basis of their ability to affect a drug's market share for a large number of consumers. The estimates of average prices for mail-order pharmacies and nonretail providers do not account for rebates. Federal facilities and purchasers who pay the best price also can receive rebates, but the estimates of average prices for federal facilities and best price do account for rebates.

a.   Conventional retail pharmacies include independent pharmacies, chain pharmacies, and food stores with pharmacies.

b.   IMS Health's data on mail-order pharmacies included information on federal mail-order facilities, which, according to the company, accounted for about 15 percent of mail-order sales. For its estimate of the average prices that mail-order pharmacies pay, CBO backed out federal facilities' purchases, assuming that those facilities obtained the same price, on average, as other federal facilities did (that is, 42 percent of the AWP).

c.   The price paid by federal facilities is based on the lowest price offered to private buyers, discounts required by federal law, and formularies. As described in Box 2 and in Congressional Budget Office, *Prices for Brand-Name Drugs Under Selected Federal Programs* (June 2005), expanding the scope of buyers who have access to the lowest price offered to private buyers would probably cause it to rise.

d.   Nonretail providers include hospitals, health maintenance organizations, clinics, home health care providers, and nursing homes.

treat chronic conditions, such substitution is more profitable.

In particular, CBO estimates, conventional pharmacies paid about 83 percent of the AWP for single-source drugs (see Table 1). Mail-order pharmacies paid no more than 78 percent, and nonretail providers paid no more than 74 percent—figures that are stated as upper bounds because the prices that CBO analyzed did not reflect all of the discounts and rebates that those providers received from manufacturers. Federal facilities paid the lowest prices, 42 percent of the AWP. By law, federal facilities have access to the lowest prices that manufacturers charge their most favored customers, and federal facilities often use formularies to negotiate additional discounts with manufacturers.

Multiple-Source Drugs

Once a brand-name drug loses its patent protection and generic versions become available, it is referred to as a multiple-source drug. When several different manufac-

turers have entered the market, pharmacies are in a strong negotiating position. In that circumstance, pharmacies, rather than PBMs, negotiate for discounted prices because they can choose which manufacturers' generic drugs to stock and, in some cases, whether to dispense the brand-name versions or the generic versions.

Although list prices such as the WAC and the AWP tend to have a consistent relationship with average transaction prices for single-source drugs and the amounts that pharmacies pay for those drugs, for generic drugs, list prices are not good predictors of pharmacies' acquisition costs. Consequently, third parties (such as health plans) making payments to pharmacies for those drugs have generally faced informational hurdles in setting payment rates that accurately reflect the pharmacies' acquisition costs. That situation will change when the AMP for drugs is made publicly available, as required by the Deficit Reduction Act of 2005. Publishing the AMP will provide greater price transparency in the retail pharmacy market.

Figure 2.

Manufacturers' Shipments of Drugs Through the Supply Chain

(Percentage of dollar sales)

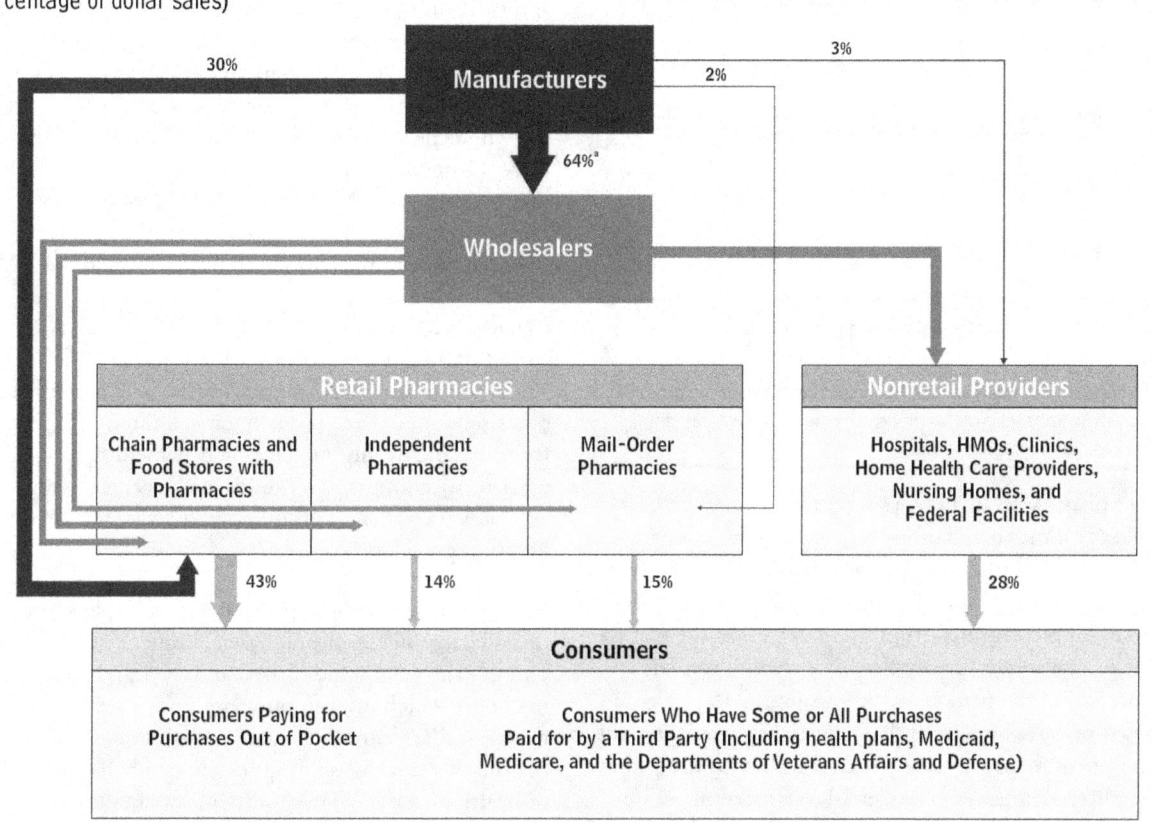

Source: Congressional Budget Office based on data from IMS Health for 2005.

Notes: HMO = health maintenance organization.

Pharmacy benefit managers (PBMs), with the exception of their mail-order pharmacies, do not take physical possession of drugs. The role of the PBMs in the payment process is shown in Figure 4.

a.   Of the 64 percent of manufacturers' shipments provided to wholesalers, the wholesalers distribute 13 percentage points' worth to chain pharmacies and food stores with pharmacies, 13 percentage points to independent pharmacies, 13 percentage points to mail-order pharmacies, and 25 percentage points to nonretail providers.

The Supply Chain

Although manufacturers sell some drugs directly to retail pharmacies and nonretail providers, most are sold to wholesalers (see Figure 2). Wholesalers decrease the number of transactions that would otherwise occur if the many retail pharmacies and nonretail providers independently ordered from hundreds of manufacturers. Retail pharmacies and nonretail providers purchase most of their products from wholesalers, but chain pharmacies and food stores with pharmacies purchase a large portion of their drugs directly from manufacturers, as they are apparently large enough to efficiently internalize aspects of the wholesale function. Nevertheless, chain pharmacies still purchase about one-quarter of their drugs (measured in dollar sales) from wholesalers, and food stores with pharmacies purchase about one-half of theirs from wholesalers (see Table 2). At the other extreme, independent pharmacies purchase 98 percent of their drugs from wholesalers.

Table 2.

Different Purchasers' Reliance on Wholesalers for Prescription Drugs

(Percentage of dollar sales)

Purchaser	Purchases from Wholesalers
Chain Pharmacies	25
Food Stores with Pharmacies	53
Independent Pharmacies	98
Mail-Order Pharmacies	85
Nonretail Providers[a]	90

Source: Congressional Budget Office based on data from IMS Health.

a. Nonretail providers include hospitals, health maintenance organizations, clinics, home health care providers, nursing homes, and federal facilities.

Retail pharmacies of all types serve about three-quarters of the consumer market for prescription drugs (see Table 3). Chain pharmacies have about half of the retail pharmacy market, and just over one-third of the entire market for prescription drugs. In recent years, the market share of mail-order pharmacies has grown—from almost 10 percent of the market in 1999 to almost 15 percent in 2005—perhaps because of the increased convenience and lower prices offered by many such facilities for drugs that treat chronic illnesses.[4] Also, employer-based plans are increasingly mandating mail order for prescription drugs that treat chronic illnesses or strongly encouraging its use through cost-sharing incentives.[5] The market share of independent pharmacies has declined— from almost 18 percent of the market in 1999 to about 14 percent in 2005.

Nonretail providers—consisting of hospitals, HMOs, clinics, home health care providers, nursing homes, and federal facilities—deliver the remaining one-fourth of prescription drugs.[6]

---

4. See Federal Trade Commission, *Pharmacy Benefit Managers: Ownership of Mail-Order Pharmacies* (August 2005), p. 18.

5. See Federal Trade Commission, *Pharmacy Benefit Managers*, p. 17. Also, as a result of the new Medicare Part D benefit, the size of the insured population that uses mail-order pharmacies for drugs that treat chronic conditions is likely to increase.

6. Drugs administered in a physician's office are included under the category of clinics.

Pricing Strategies and Measures

The prices paid to manufacturers for prescription drugs depend both on the competitive conditions in the market as well as on the bargaining power of purchasers. There are three price measures that are important in understanding the payment system for prescription drugs in the retail pharmacy market: the average manufacturer price, the wholesale acquisition cost, and the average wholesale price. Generally, in the retail pharmacy market for single-source drugs, the AMP is the price paid to manufacturers, the WAC approximates the price paid to wholesalers, and the price paid to pharmacies is often based on the AWP.

Pricing Strategies

The structure of competition differs dramatically for single-source drugs and generic drugs. The manufacturer of a single-source drug usually faces limited competition from therapeutically similar brand-name drugs on the market. By contrast, the producer of a generic drug usually faces several competitors offering what are nearly identical products.[7]

Single-Source Drugs. Manufacturers of single-source drugs charge different purchasers different prices based on both the volume purchased and the purchaser's ability to choose which drug to purchase from a set of therapeutically similar drugs. Nonretail providers and mail-order pharmacies (managing drug benefits on behalf of PBMs or health plans) have the ability to systematically favor one brand-name drug over another and therefore tend to pay lower prices for brand-name drugs than conventional pharmacies do. Conventional pharmacies tend to fill prescriptions for single-source drugs as written by the doctor and therefore lack the ability to favor one single-source drug over another. When pharmacies do contact doctors to change prescriptions, they may be acting on behalf of PBMs or health plans using formularies to manage drug spending, in which case, any rebates would go to the PBMs or the health plans and not the pharmacies.

Nonretail providers and mail-order pharmacies that buy directly from manufacturers can simply negotiate lower prices for choosing the manufacturers' drugs over competing drugs. However, as mentioned, about two-thirds of manufacturers' sales are directed through wholesalers. But that arrangement does not prevent purchasers from

---

7. Most generic drugs are rated by the Food and Drug Administration as bioequivalent to the brand-name product.

Table 3.

U.S. Sales of Prescription Drugs and Sellers' Market Shares, 1999 and 2005

	1999		2005	
	Sales (Billions of dollars)	Market Share (Percent)	Sales (Billions of dollars)	Market Share (Percent)
Retail				
Chain Pharmacies	53.6	38.9	88.2	35.0
Mail-Order Pharmacies	13.2	9.6	36.9	14.7
Independent Pharmacies	24.4	17.7	34.4	13.6
Food Stores with Pharmacies	12.7	9.2	21.3	8.5
Subtotal, Retail	103.8	75.4	180.8	71.8
Nonretail				
Nonfederal Hospitals	15.3	11.1	26.0	10.3
Clinics	8.7	6.3	24.8	9.9
Nursing Homes	3.9	2.8	12.0	4.8
Federal Facilities	2.2	1.6	3.6	1.4
Home Health Care Providers	1.5	1.1	2.4	0.9
HMOs	1.6	1.2	1.5	0.6
Miscellaneous Facilities	0.6	0.4	0.8	0.3
Subtotal, Nonretail	33.8	24.6	71.1	28.2
Total U.S. Market	**137.7**	**100.0**	**251.8**	**100.0**

Source: Congressional Budget office based on data from IMS Health for 1999 and 2005 (the most recent data available); see
www.imshealth.com/ims/portal/front/articleC/0,2777,6599_73915261_77141536,00.html.

Note: HMO = health maintenance organization.

obtaining lower net prices. Manufacturers frequently pay rebates directly to purchasers on the basis of the volume of drugs they purchase over a period of time. A demonstrated ability to switch patients to a particular company's drug, evidenced by an increase in the volume sold to a purchaser's customers, may be rewarded with a higher rebate. In that case, the purchaser's net price is the amount paid to the wholesaler minus the rebate. The rebate is an "off-invoice" pricing adjustment; that is, it is not reflected in the wholesaler's invoice price, having been negotiated privately between the manufacturer and the purchaser. Obtaining information about the size of such rebates and which purchasers get them is usually not possible, so most of the prices analyzed by CBO in this paper do not include them.[8]

Manufacturers also pay rebates to PBMs working on behalf of health plans. PBMs determine which drugs are therapeutically similar.[9] Then, for such brand-name drugs with several close substitutes, PBMs negotiate with manufacturers for rebates in return for placing the manufacturers' drugs on their formularies or giving the drugs

preferential placement on their formularies. PBMs can give preferential treatment to manufacturers' drugs by, for example, charging a lower copayment for the preferred drugs than for other (nonpreferred) drugs that are therapeutically similar. The health plans' patients may then have access to only the identified drugs (in what is known as a closed formulary) or may have access to nearly all prescription drugs but at different levels of cost sharing (in what is known as an open formulary).

Generic Drugs. With generic drugs, conventional pharmacies and wholesalers, in addition to nonretail providers

8. For further discussion of pricing in the pharmaceutical industry, see Congressional Budget Office, *How Increased Competition from Generic Drugs Has Affected Prices and Returns in the Pharmaceutical Industry* (July 1998), Chapter 3; and Richard G. Frank, "Prescription Drug Prices: Why Do Some Pay More Than Others Do?" *Health Affairs*, vol. 20, no. 2 (2001), pp. 115–128.

9. A pharmacy and therapeutics committee, made up of physicians and pharmacists, usually determines which drugs within the same therapeutic class are close substitutes.

Figure 3.

Measures of Prices in the Retail Pharmacy Market

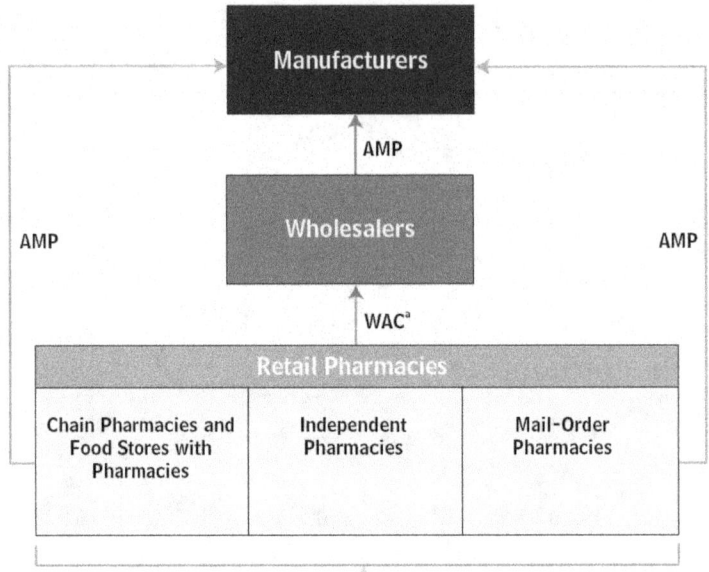

Source: Congressional Budget Office.

Notes: AMP = average manufacturer price; WAC = wholesale acquisition cost; AWP = average wholesale price.

  The AMP is an average of actual transaction prices. In contrast, the WAC and the AWP are list prices, like a sticker price in the automobile industry.

  The role of the pharmacy benefit managers in the payment process is shown in Figure 4.

a. The WAC approximates what conventional retail pharmacies pay wholesalers for single-source brand-name drugs. It does not approximate what retail pharmacies pay wholesalers for multiple-source drugs.

and mail-order pharmacies, choose which versions to stock. Consequently, those purchasers are able to negotiate lower prices from manufacturers. Chain pharmacies that purchase large volumes of generic drugs may negotiate lower prices than other purchasers of smaller volumes. PBMs, working on behalf of health plans, do not choose which generic drugs to dispense and so are not in a position to negotiate lower prices with manufacturers.[10]

Price Measures

Of the three pricing measures that are important in understanding the payment system for prescription drugs in the retail pharmacy market, only one is an average of actual transaction prices: the average manufacturer price. The other two prices are list prices that are something like the sticker price on a car: the wholesale acquisition cost and the average wholesale price. (See Figure 3.)

---

10. An exception would be a mail-order pharmacy owned by a PBM.

Box 1.

The Average Manufacturer Price Is to Be Made Publicly Available

Currently, the average manufacturer price (AMP) for prescription drugs is not publicly available. That situation will change when the Centers for Medicare & Medicaid Services (CMS) publicly posts AMPs for both generic and brand-name drugs, as required under the Deficit Reduction Act, which the agency expects to do late in the spring of 2007.[1] The AMPs are being made publicly available in part to help implement Medicaid's new payment rate for multiple-source drugs, which was changed by the Deficit Reduction Act. That rate will be equal to 250 percent of the lowest AMP among generic drugs and their brand-name counterparts with the same active ingredients, dosage form, and strength. As part of implementing the new payment rate, CMS has issued a proposed rule that includes a new definition of the AMP.[2]

AMPs do not reflect all pharmacies' acquisition costs because they do not include wholesalers' markups. Further, AMPs are average prices across all retail pharmacy channels and include discounts that may not be available to all pharmacies. Nonetheless, making AMPs public may help inform payments to pharmacies by third-party payers and particularly the upper limits that payers place on payments to pharmacies for multiple-source drugs. Making AMPs publicly available may also enable insurance companies, employers, and cash customers to determine whether they are paying appropriate amounts for particular drugs—thus, overall, bringing greater price transparency to the retail pharmacy market. This additional pricing information could lower what pharmacies and wholesalers are paid for prescription drugs. In addition, to the extent that different pharmacies currently pay different prices for the same prescription drugs, making AMPs public could narrow the range of prices that pharmacies pay.

1. See Centers for Medicare & Medicaid Services, "Medicaid Drug Pricing Regulation Proposed" (fact sheet, December 15, 2006), available at www.cms.hhs.gov/apps/media/fact_sheets.asp.

2. The proposed rule is available at www.cms.hhs.gov/MedicaidGenInfo/downloads/AMP2238P.pdf.

The average manufacturer price is the average price paid by wholesalers to manufacturers or by retail pharmacies that buy directly from manufacturers for drugs distributed through retail pharmacies. It reflects all rebates paid by manufacturers to wholesalers and to retail pharmacies. It does not include rebates paid by manufacturers to PBMs, Medicaid, or to other third-party payers. Manufacturers are required to report the AMP to the Centers for Medicare & Medicaid Services, which uses it to calculate the rebates that the manufacturers are required to pay to state Medicaid programs for sales to beneficiaries.[11] Currently, the AMP is confidential, but, as required under the Deficit Reduction Act of 2005, it will be made publicly available by CMS, probably in the spring of 2007 (see Box 1).

The wholesale acquisition cost is a publicly available list price for sales by manufacturers to wholesalers. Manufacturers report the WAC to publications such as Thomson Micromedex's *Red Book* and First DataBank's *Blue Book*.[12] The WAC does not represent actual transaction prices, and it is not, despite its name, what wholesalers pay for drugs. However, for single-source brand-name drugs, the WAC approximates what retail pharmacies pay wholesalers. Perhaps because the WAC is a publicly available price that closely approximates what retail pharmacies pay for drugs, negotiated rebates for brand-name drugs between PBMs and manufacturers are sometimes based on it.[13]

11. The savings from those rebate payments are shared with the federal government.

12. This paper relies on the WAC for drugs reported in Thomson Micromedex's *Red Book*.

13. See Federal Trade Commission, *Pharmacy Benefit Managers*, p. 50.

For generic drugs, the WAC does not approximate what retail pharmacies pay wholesalers. Because third parties' payments to pharmacies for generic drugs are often based on list prices such as the WAC, a manufacturer has an incentive to set a high WAC and increase the spread between what pharmacies pay wholesalers and the payments that the pharmacies receive—thereby encouraging pharmacies to dispense its generic drugs. (While health plans are aware that the WAC greatly exceeds the pharmacies' acquisition costs for generic drugs, they have only limited information on the actual costs.) By contrast, because pharmacies do not choose which single-source drugs to dispense, a manufacturer has little incentive to attempt to increase the spread between what pharmacies pay wholesalers and the payment that pharmacies receive from health plans. Perhaps that is partly why the WAC for single-source drugs closely approximates what retail pharmacies pay wholesalers.

The average wholesale price is a publicly available list price for sales by wholesalers to pharmacies and nonretail providers—again, reported in publications such as Thomson Micromedex's *Red Book* and First DataBank's *Blue Book*. The AWP does not represent actual transaction prices, and it is not, as its name suggests, what wholesalers charge for drugs. According to First Data-Bank, the AWP data that it publishes are intended to represent an average of wholesalers' list prices. However, a class action lawsuit has been brought against the company alleging that it began relying exclusively on information provided by the wholesaler McKesson as the basis for its published AWP data and did not survey any other wholesalers.[14] This paper relies upon AWP data reported

by Thomson Micromedex, which, according to the company, are reported by manufacturers.

The AWP is often used as a basis for payment to retail pharmacies by, for example, the Medicaid program, PBMs, and health plans. For example, a PBM's or health plan's "typical" payment rate to a pharmacy for a single-source brand-name drug in 2003 was the AWP minus 15 percent plus a $2 dispensing fee.[15] A PBM's payment rate to a pharmacy for a multiple-source drug can be based on the AWP of all brand-name and generic drugs that are chemically equivalent.

The Roles of Pharmacy Benefit Managers and Pharmacies

PBMs manage pharmacy benefits on behalf of their clients, which include health plans, HMOs, and self-insured employer-based plans. Their primary services include claims administration, reviews of drug utilization, formulary management, and negotiated pricing arrangements with drug manufacturers and the PBMs' network of retail pharmacies.[16] One expert has estimated that the three largest PBMs (Caremark RX, Medco, and Express Scripts) together manage more than one-third of all drug sales in the retail pharmacy market.[17] Pharmacies dispense prescriptions to consumers and perform other services such as checking for drug interactions and proper dosage levels. Pharmacies can also help to administer PBMs' formularies.

Pharmacy Benefit Managers
PBMs play a key role in negotiating the final price that manufacturers and pharmacies receive on a prescription drug sale. Manufacturers set their price to wholesalers and pharmacies with an eye toward the availability of other close substitutes on the market, keeping in mind

---

14. The lawsuit also alleges that First DataBank and McKesson illegally conspired to increase the spread between what pharmacies pay wholesalers and the reimbursement that pharmacies receive from health plans by increasing AWPs from a standard of 20 percent above WACs to 25 percent above. If a proposed settlement is approved and ordered by the Boston district court, First DataBank will reduce its AWPs to 20 percent above WACs and will discontinue publishing AWPs within two years of the effective date of the final court order. See Kathryn Phelps, "First DataBank AWP Settlement Pressures Pharmacies to Change Payment," *The Pink Sheet*, October 16, 2006, pp. 13–14; Barbara Martinez, "Book Value: How Quiet Moves by a Publisher Sway Billions in Drug Spending," *Wall Street Journal*, October 6, 2006, pp. A1 and A12; and Memorandum from First DataBank to Customers, "AWP Communications Re: First DataBank's *Blue Book* AWP Data," October 5, 2006, available at www.firstdatabank.com/support/rcs/communications/awp/.

15. See Novartis Pharmaceuticals Corporation, *Pharmacy Benefit Report: Facts & Figures* (2004), p. 16.

16. For more detailed descriptions of how PBMs work, see Kaiser Family Foundation, *The Role of PBMs in Managing Drug Costs: Implications for a Medicare Drug Benefit* (January 2000). See also D. Kreling and others, *Assessment of the Impact of Pharmacy Benefit Managers* (Health Care Financing Administration, National Technical Information Service, Publication No. PB97-103683, September 1996).

17. Robert Atlas, "The Role of PBMs in Implementing the Medicare Prescription Drug Benefit," *Health Affairs*, Web Exclusive, October 28, 2004, pp. W4-504–W4-515.

Figure 4.

Flow of Funds for Single-Source Brand-Name Drugs Purchased at a Retail Pharmacy and Managed by a Pharmacy Benefit Manager for an Employer's Health Plan

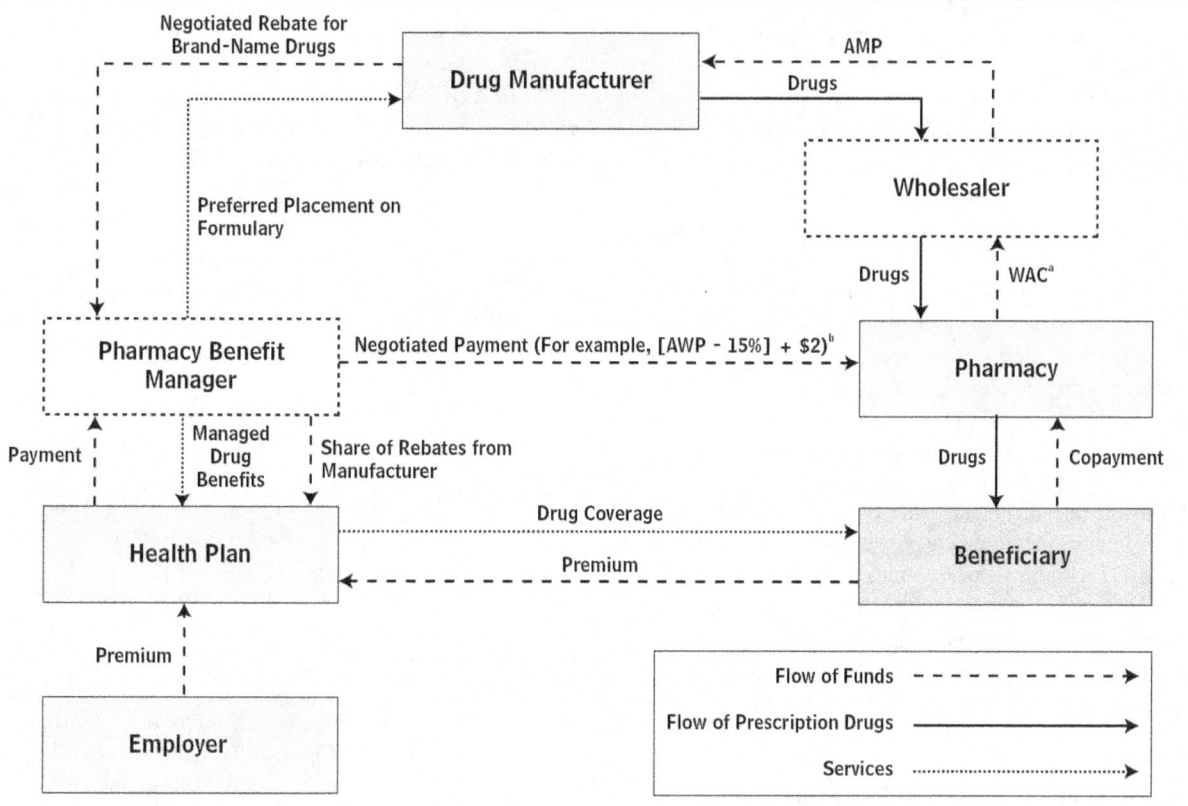

Source: Congressional Budget Office.

Note: AMP = average manufacturer price; WAC = wholesale acquisition cost; AWP = average wholesale price.

a.   The WAC is a list price that approximates what conventional pharmacies pay wholesalers for single-source brand-name drugs.

b.   Based on Novartis Pharmaceuticals Corporation, *Pharmacy Benefit Report: Facts & Figures* (2004), p. 16.

that they will pay rebates to certain types of purchasers, such as a PBM working on behalf of a health plan (see Figure 4).[18] Thus, the price paid by wholesalers and pharmacies that buy directly from the manufacturers is not the final net price received by manufacturers. That final net price received by the manufacturer is the AMP minus any rebates paid to the PBM.

The formulary is one of the main cost-containment mechanisms used by a PBM. How much copayments are, whether or not all drugs are covered, and how much more beneficiaries must pay for nonpreferred drugs are determined in discussions between the PBM and the health plan or employer. Other contractual mechanisms that affect the cost of the drug benefit include the share of rebates that the health plan will receive, the size of any administrative fee paid to the PBM, and the price that

18. Other types of purchasers that get rebate payments include Medicaid; health plans that internalize the PBM function; and nonretail providers, including hospitals, HMOs, and clinics.

the health plan will pay for prescription drugs (which can differ from what the PBM pays the pharmacy).[19]

In negotiating with a manufacturer, the PBM has the greatest leverage for brand-name drugs with close substitutes available on the market. Rebates by the manufacturer can come in two forms: formulary payments, which are in exchange for favorable placement on a formulary, and market-share payments, which are based on the market share that the manufacturer's drug receives relative to its close competitors. The type and size of rebates can vary over a product's life. For example, market-share payments are usually not provided for a new breakthrough drug. And formulary payments are very small or perhaps nonexistent for such a drug because there are no alternatives on the market. As other similar drugs are introduced on the market, the manufacturer may start to negotiate formulary and market-share payments. The manufacturer will usually stop making rebate payments to the PBM once a generic drug becomes available.[20]

Manufacturers also make other types of payments to PBMs in addition to rebate payments. For example, manufacturers commonly pay a fee to PBMs for the service of administering formularies. Such fees are frequently equal to about 3 percent of wholesale list prices. Other types of payments cover programs such as ones promoting the use of one therapeutically similar drug over another.[21]

Pharmacies

Pharmacies do not have much leverage to negotiate with manufacturers for discounts on single-source brand-name drugs.[22] Pharmacies stock a wide range of single-source

drugs so that they are prepared to immediately fill most prescriptions on demand. However, they do have leverage to negotiate with manufacturers for discounts on multiple-source drugs because they can choose which manufacturers' drugs to stock and dispense. When the beneficiary of a health plan managed by a PBM goes to a pharmacy to purchase a drug and presents his or her card associated with the plan, the pharmacist can process the claim immediately using technology that determines whether the drug is on the PBM's formulary, whether it is a preferred brand-name drug, and what the copayment is. In those ways, the pharmacist administers the PBM's formulary—along with performing other services such as checking for drug interactions and proper dosage. Yet even when the pharmacist helps to administer the formulary, any rebate payment for a single-source drug goes to the PBM (or health plan), not the pharmacy.

PBMs' Negotiated Payments to Pharmacies. PBMs negotiate with pharmacies over payments for prescription drugs purchased by the associated health plans' patients. Those negotiated payments have two separate components: reimbursements for the drugs and payments for the dispensing service. The component composed of reimbursements by PBMs and third-party payers such as Medicaid for the cost of the single-source brand-name drugs is usually determined using a formula based on the AWP.[23] Pharmacies may be willing to accept lower total payments in exchange for the greater volume of sales that can come from joining PBMs' pharmacy networks.

Mail-Order Pharmacies. The majority of mail-order pharmacies are owned by PBMs, and a number of large chain pharmacies also own mail-order pharmacies.[24] Mail-order pharmacies may have lower dispensing costs than conventional pharmacies do and, when working on behalf of PBMs or health plans, can help to improve compliance with formularies. In the mail-order setting, the pharmacist has more time to contact a physician and attempt to obtain permission to switch a prescription from a drug not on the formulary to a less expensive drug that is on the formulary. Furthermore, a large share of

19. Some contracts vary the rebate share—for example, the more controls in the benefit (in terms of increasing the cost sharing for nonpreferred drugs and limiting the formulary to fewer drugs), the larger the share of rebate payments the health plan is likely to obtain. For more details, see Federal Trade Commission, *Pharmacy Benefit Managers*, pp. 57–60.

20. See Federal Trade Commission, *Pharmacy Benefit Managers*, pp. 50–55.

21. See Federal Trade Commission, *Pharmacy Benefit Managers*, pp. 55–56.

22. Pharmacies do not benefit from the rebates that manufacturers give to PBMs. At the same time, pharmacies that do a better job of dispensing generic drugs when those drugs provide an alternative to brand-name drugs and promoting compliance with PBMs' formularies may obtain more favorable payment rates from the PBMs.

23. Payment rates for multiple-source drugs are a bit more complicated—though they also involve a payment for ingredient costs and a dispensing fee. Those rates are explained below.

24. See The Health Strategies Consultancy LLC, "Follow the Pill: Understanding the U.S. Commercial Pharmaceutical Supply Chain" (prepared for the Kaiser Family Foundation, March 2005), p. 13.

mail-order prescriptions are for chronic conditions, so a substitution can affect not only the prescription currently being dispensed but also many to come in the future, making the practice more profitable than it might otherwise be. Finally, PBMs may choose to establish mail-order pharmacies because by purchasing drugs for them, the PBMs obtain more information on the acquisition costs (which is particularly important for multiple-source drugs) that they can then use in their negotiations over payments with their retail pharmacy networks.

Single-Source Brand-Name Drugs

CBO analyzed the prices paid for a sample of single-source drugs at different points in the pharmaceutical supply chain. The sample—which consisted of drugs in oral solid dosage forms (tablets and capsules)—constituted about 40 percent of total U.S. sales of prescription drugs in 2003, including a majority of the top sellers in the retail pharmacy market and their close substitutes.[25] According to CBO's estimates, the AMP for the drugs in the sample in the fourth quarter of calendar year 2003 was about 79 percent of the AWP, on average.[26]

The prices paid by retail pharmacies and nonretail providers are based on data from IMS Health's National Sales Perspectives, which compiles information on dollar and unit sales from manufacturers, wholesalers, and chain warehouses for each of the different types of purchasers (that is, independent pharmacies, chain pharmacies, food stores with pharmacies, mail-order pharmacies, home health care providers, nursing homes, HMOs with pharmacies, nonfederal hospitals, clinics, and federal facilities). Using those data, for each of the different types of purchasers, CBO calculated weighted average prices as a percentage of the AWP on the basis of the quantities of those drugs sold in the United States:

■ Those prices are average prices paid for drugs by retail pharmacies and nonretail providers to their suppliers, which could be wholesalers, chain warehouses (in the case of chain pharmacies and food stores with pharmacies), or manufacturers.

■ The prices do not reflect rebates paid by manufacturers to mail-order pharmacies or nonretail providers.

■ However, they can capture a form of discount called charge-backs, which are handled through the wholesalers.[27]

Prices Paid by Retail Pharmacies

As described, independent pharmacies purchase about 98 percent of their drugs from wholesalers, so the average price paid by independent pharmacies largely represents the average price paid to wholesalers. Chain pharmacies purchase about three-quarters of their drugs from their own chain warehouses, and food stores with pharmacies purchase about half of their drugs from their own chain warehouses. Prices collected from chain warehouses most likely do not reflect market prices, which occur in arm's-length transactions between independent parties, but instead represent transfer prices used for the purpose of internal accounting. So average prices paid by chain pharmacies and food stores with pharmacies should be viewed with caution.

By CBO's estimates, the average price paid by conventional retail outlets (that is, independent pharmacies, chain pharmacies, and food stores with pharmacies) was 82 percent to 83 percent of the AWP (see Table 4). The average price for conventional retail outlets was roughly the same as the WAC. Although the average prices calculated from IMS Health's data do not reflect rebates paid by manufacturers to wholesalers and retail pharmacies, conventional retail outlets generally do not receive rebates for single-source drugs—as they tend to dispense prescriptions as written by physicians rather than actively steering drug purchases to certain manufacturers' drugs.

Wholesalers retain the difference between the price that they pay to manufacturers and the price that retail pharmacies pay them, the wholesalers. On the basis of that difference between the AMP and the average amount paid by retail pharmacies, the amount attributable to the wholesale function (performed by wholesalers or chain or food store warehouses) was about 3 percent of the AWP, on average, CBO estimates.[28]

---

25. See the appendix for a description of the data on drug prices that CBO used, as well as an explanation of the methodology used to calculate average prices relative to list prices.

26. Results for other quarters in calendar year 2003 are similar.

27. Manufacturers negotiate discounted prices with some purchasers who buy through wholesalers. The wholesalers deliver the drugs at the discounted price, inform the manufacturers ("charging back" the discount), and then are reimbursed by the manufacturers. See Congressional Budget Office, *How Increased Competition from Generic Drugs Has Affected Prices and Returns in the Pharmaceutical Industry* (July 1998), pp. 24–25.

28. That amount will vary among purchasers depending partly upon the type of wholesale services provided.

Table 4.

Average Prices for Single-Source Brand-Name Drugs Relative to the Average Wholesale Price, at Different Points in the Supply Chain

	Are Rebates That Are Not Reflected in the Price Shown Likely?	Average Price as a Percentage of AWP
Price Measures		
Average wholesale price	Not a transaction price	100
Wholesale acquisition cost	Not a transaction price	82
Average manufacturer price	Price includes rebates to retail pharmacies and wholesalers but not to third-party payers	79
Retail Pharmacies		
Conventional pharmacies		
Independent	No	82
Chain[a]	No	82
Food stores[a]	No	83
All conventional pharmacies	No	83
Mail-order[b]	Yes	No More Than 78
All Retail Pharmacies	**Yes**	**No More Than 82**
Nonretail Providers		
Federal facilities	No	42[c]
Nonretail providers excluding federal facilities		
Home health care providers	Yes	No More Than 83
Nursing homes	Yes	No More Than 80
HMOs	Yes	No More Than 79
Nonfederal hospitals	Yes	No More Than 71
Clinics	Yes	No More Than 69
All nonretail (nonfederal) facilities	Yes	No More Than 74
All Nonretail Providers	**Yes**	**No More Than 66**
Best Price	No	64

Source: Congressional Budget Office (CBO) based on data from IMS Health for the fourth quarter of 2003.

Notes: AWP = average wholesale price; HMO = health maintenance organization.

The sample—which consisted of drugs in oral solid dosage forms (tablets and capsules)—constituted about 40 percent of total U.S. sales of prescription drugs in 2003, including most top sellers in the retail pharmacy market and their close substitutes.

Mail-order pharmacies and nonretail providers can receive rebates from manufacturers on the basis of their ability to affect a drug's market share. The estimates of average prices for mail-order pharmacies and nonretail providers do not account for rebates. Federal facilities and purchasers who pay the best price also can receive rebates, but the estimates of average prices for federal facilities and best price do account for rebates.

a. Chain pharmacies and food stores with pharmacies purchase a large portion of their drugs from their own chain warehouses instead of wholesalers. The chain warehouses' prices probably do not reflect market prices, which occur in arm's-length transactions between independent parties but, instead, represent transfer prices for the purpose of internal accounting. Consequently, the average prices obtained from IMS's data may not reflect what the pharmacies actually paid manufacturers.

b. IMS Health's data on mail-order pharmacies included information on federal mail-order facilities, which, according to the company, accounted for about 15 percent of mail-order sales. For its estimate of the average prices that mail-order pharmacies pay, CBO backed out federal facilities' purchases, assuming that those facilities obtained the same price, on average, as other federal facilities did (that is, 42 percent of the AWP).

c. The price paid by federal facilities is based on the lowest price offered to private buyers, discounts required by federal law, and formularies. As described in Box 2 and in Congressional Budget Office, *Prices for Brand-Name Drugs Under Selected Federal Programs* (June 2005), expanding the scope of buyers who have access to the lowest price offered to private buyers would probably cause it to rise.

The price that mail-order pharmacies paid to wholesalers was no more than 78 percent, on average, according to CBO's estimates.[29] Mail-order pharmacies may receive rebates from manufacturers on some of their drug purchases, which the data do not include, so that estimate constitutes an upper bound. The lower prices obtained by mail-order pharmacies may reflect, in part, their greater ability to promote compliance with formularies compared with conventional pharmacies' ability.

Prices Paid by Nonretail Providers

The average prices paid by nonretail providers do not reflect rebates paid by manufacturers to providers (with the exception of federal facilities). Nonretail providers may receive rebates from manufacturers because the providers can choose which drugs from sets of therapeutically similar drugs to dispense in their facilities. Because rebates are not reflected in the prices nonretail providers pay to wholesalers, CBO's estimates of the prices they pay represent an upper bound, and the relative ranking of the prices paid by the different nonretail providers could change once the rebates from the manufacturers to the nonretail providers are accounted for.

The average prices paid by nonretail providers are generally less than those of conventional retail outlets. That finding is consistent with the notion that purchasers are rewarded for their ability to influence the choices about prescriptions for a large number of patients. In CBO's estimates, the average price paid by nonretail providers ranged from no more than 83 percent of the AWP for home health care providers to no more than 42 percent for federal facilities (see Table 4). The average price paid by all nonretail providers was no more than 66 percent of the AWP.

With federal facilities excluded from the calculation, that average price for nonretail facilities was no more than 74 percent of the AWP. Federal facilities include hospitals run by the Department of Veterans Affairs (VA) and the Department of Defense (DoD), which have access to fed-

eral prices (for example, prices on the Federal Supply Schedule and federal ceiling prices) that, by law, are at least as low as the prices manufacturers charge their most-favored commercial customers under comparable terms and conditions. In addition to those already low prices, VA and DoD use their formularies to negotiate even greater discounts with manufacturers. Because the discounts are often processed through the wholesalers that supply the agencies, the majority of those discounts are reflected in CBO's estimates of the average prices paid by federal facilities.[30]

The distribution of rebates is unknown, but the best price, or the lowest price paid by any private-sector purchaser of a drug, including all discounts and rebates, as reported to CMS, is known.[31] The best price is used to calculate the rebates that manufacturers are required to give to state governments for sales of brand-name drugs to Medicaid beneficiaries. Manufacturers must report it to CMS in order to be paid for those drugs. Some private-sector purchasers pay higher prices as a result of the best-price provision in Medicaid's rebate program (see Box 2).

The average best price as a percentage of the AWP provides a lower bound for the price that mail-order pharmacies and nonretail providers (excluding federal facilities) pay for brand-name drugs once rebates from manufacturers are taken into account. (It is unlikely that any of the purchasers reach that lower bound because no purchaser gets the best price on every drug.) In CBO's estimates, the best price was 64 percent of the AWP, on average—thus, 5 to 19 percentage points below the average prices paid by mail-order pharmacies and nonretail (nonfederal) providers.

---

29. IMS Health's data on mail-order pharmacies included information on federal mail-order facilities, which, according to the company, accounted for about 15 percent of mail-order sales. For its estimate of the average prices that mail-order pharmacies pay, CBO backed out federal facilities' purchases, assuming that those facilities obtained the same price, on average, as other federal facilities did (that is, 42 percent of the AWP).

---

30. If access to the lowest private-sector prices was extended to other purchasers through regulation, manufacturers would probably raise those prices. See Box 2, and for more information about the prices paid by federal facilities, see Congressional Budget Office, *Prices for Brand-Name Drugs Under Selected Federal Programs* (June 2005).

31. In a review that the Government Accountability Office conducted, it "found considerable variation in the methods that manufacturers used to determine best price. . . ." See Government Accountability Office, *Medicaid Drug Rebate Program: Inadequate Oversight Raises Concerns About Rebates Paid to States*, GAO-05-102 (February 2005), p. 15.

Box 2.
Medicaid's Rebate Program

The best price, or the lowest price paid by any private-sector purchaser of a drug, including all discounts and rebates, is used to calculate the rebates that manufacturers are required by law to give to state governments for sales of brand-name drugs to Medicaid beneficiaries. Manufacturers must report the price to the Centers for Medicare & Medicaid Services in order to be paid for those drugs.

Rather than extending their best prices to the entire Medicaid market, firms have frequently chosen to raise their best prices.[1] Medicaid's rebate is equal to the greater of 15.1 percent of the average manufacturer price (AMP) or the difference between the best price and the AMP. In 1991, when the Medicaid rebate program was first implemented, the best price was, on average, 36 percent below the AMP for brand-name drugs. Since 1996, the best price has been a little more than 15 percent below the AMP, on average—roughly the level at which the best-price provision is triggered.

For a brief period in 1991 and part of 1992, prices on the Federal Supply Schedule were included in the calculation of the best price; and during that period, many of the Federal Supply Schedule prices increased.[2] Legislation was then enacted to exclude Federal Supply Schedule prices from the calculation of the best price. More recently, to help Medicare Part D plans obtain lower prices, their negotiated prices were excluded from Medicaid's best-price provision under the Medicare Modernization Act.

The effect that the best-price provision has on the private-sector price of a drug (that is, the tendency to raise it) is greater the larger Medicaid's market share is. On average, the effect of the best-price provision on private-sector prices is likely to decline as Medicaid's market share is reduced by the movement of Medicaid beneficiaries to the new Medicare Part D drug benefit.

---

1. See Congressional Budget Office, *The Rebate Medicaid Receives on Brand-Name Prescription Drugs* (June 21, 2005).

2. See General Accounting Office, *Medicaid: Changes in Drug Prices Paid by VA and DOD Since Enactment of Rebate Provisions*, GAO/HRD-91-139 (September 1991).

A Hypothetical Example

An August 2005 report by the Federal Trade Commission (FTC) examined rebates from manufacturers to PBMs, for which the agency subpoenaed data and documents.[32] The FTC found that in 2002 the average rebate per brand-name prescription to PBMs was $5.22 and that in 2003 it was $6.34 (or about 6 percent of the average cost of a single-source prescription in CBO's sample at the

AWP). In the study, each PBM's top 25 brand-name drugs accounted for about 70 percent of rebate payments.

By combining results from CBO's sample of single-source drugs with results from the FTC report, a hypothetical example can be constructed. Consider a situation in which an independent pharmacy bought a drug from a wholesaler and sold it to a consumer with a drug benefit managed by a PBM (see Figure 5):

---

32. Federal Trade Commission, *Pharmacy Benefit Managers*, p. 47.

Figure 5.

Hypothetical Example of Payments for a Single-Source Prescription

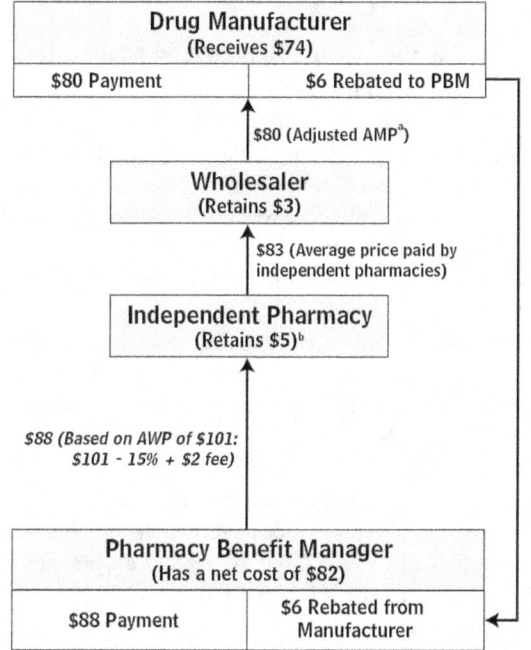

Source: Congressional Budget Office (CBO) based on its estimates of average prices (see Table 4); Federal Trade Commission, *Pharmacy Benefit Managers: Ownership of Mail-Order Pharmacies* (August 2005); and Novartis Pharmaceuticals Corporation, *Pharmacy Benefit Report: Facts & Figures* (2004), p. 16.

Notes: PBM = pharmacy benefit manager; AMP = average manufacturer price; AWP = average wholesale price.

In this example, an independent pharmacy buys a single-source prescription from a wholesaler and sells it to a consumer who has a drug benefit overseen by a PBM.

In CBO's sample, covering the fourth quarter of 2003, $101 is the average cost of a single-source brand-name drug at the AWP.

The estimate of $6 for rebates and other payments was drawn from the Federal Trade Commission's report.

a. Adjusted to remove mail-order sales from the AMP.

b. CBO used AWP data purchased from Thomson Micromedex. If other sources had higher AWPs on average, and CBO had used them, the estimated payment to the retail pharmacy would have been higher, and the estimated amount that it retained would have been higher as well.

■ On average, the wholesaler would pay the manufacturer a bit more than the AMP for a drug distributed through an independent pharmacy, or about $80, for a single-source prescription in CBO's sample.[33]

■ The independent pharmacy would pay the wholesaler about $83 for the prescription. The difference between what the wholesaler paid the manufacturer (roughly the AMP) and what the pharmacy paid the wholesaler is the amount retained by the wholesaler, or in this example about $3.

■ According to a Novartis report, a "typical" payment rate to a pharmacy for a single-source prescription under a managed drug benefit in 2003 was the AWP minus 15 percent plus a $2 dispensing fee.[34] The average cost of a single-source prescription in CBO's sample at the AWP was about $101, so the pharmacy would receive about $88. (Any copayment made by the beneficiary would contribute toward that $88 total, with the PBM paying the balance). The difference between what the pharmacy paid the wholesaler and what the pharmacy receives (the AWP minus 15 percent plus $2 for the dispensing fee) is the amount retained by the pharmacy, or in this example about $5.[35]

■ The manufacturer keeps the amount paid to it by the wholesaler (roughly the AMP) minus any rebates paid to the PBM. According to the FTC report, rebates and other payments from manufacturers to PBMs averaged about $6 per prescription in 2003. So an approximation of the amount retained by the manufacturer would be $74 ($80 minus $6).

33. The AMP includes manufacturers' sales to mail-order pharmacies, which tend to get lower prices than conventional pharmacies on single-source drugs. Wholesalers may pay manufacturers a bit more than the AMP, on average, for single-source drugs distributed to conventional pharmacies. Taking the results from Table 4 as reflecting the price that mail-order pharmacies receive relative to independent pharmacies and accounting for mail-order pharmacies' share of the retail market implies that removing mail-order sales from the AMP would increase the prescription cost from $79 to $80.

34. Novartis Pharmaceuticals Corporation, *Pharmacy Benefit Report: Facts & Figures* (2004), p. 16.

35. CBO used AWP data purchased from Thomson Micromedex. If other sources had higher AWPs, on average, and CBO had used them, then estimated payments to the retail pharmacy would have been higher, and the estimated amount that it retained would have been higher as well.

■ Overall, the independent pharmacy retained 6 percent of the payment made by the PBM to the pharmacy, the manufacturer received 84 percent, the wholesaler retained 3 percent, and the remaining 7 percent consisted of rebates and other payments from the manufacturer to the PBM. Rebate payments from manufacturers are usually shared between the PBMs and health plans. Such percentages are only illustrative because among various drugs, pharmacies, manufacturers, wholesalers, and PBMs, the estimated amounts retained by each party will vary widely.

Cash Customers

According to the FTC report, customers without insurance paid conventional pharmacies 15 percent more for single-source brand-name drugs than customers with insurance paid.[36] Furthermore, cash customers without insurance do not benefit from the rebate system. Thus, cash customers (such as the uninsured) pay among the highest prices for such drugs.

Multiple-Source Drugs

Once a brand-name drug loses patent protection and generic versions become available, both the brand-name drug and its generic counterparts are referred to as multiple-source drugs. The pricing dynamics differ markedly for generic drugs. First, the markets are much more competitive than the ones for brand-name drugs. Once several manufacturers of a generic drug have entered a market, prices for the drug quickly fall to a fraction of the price of the brand-name counterpart.[37] Further, in the market for generic drugs, wholesalers, retail pharmacies, and mail-order pharmacies (rather than PBMs) have the leverage to negotiate with manufacturers for lower prices. Whereas PBMs choose which single-source drugs to give preferred placement on their formularies on the basis of the outcome of negotiations, it is the pharmacists who

choose which generic drugs to stock and dispense when multiple versions are available.[38] Chain pharmacies that purchase large volumes of generic drugs may negotiate lower prices than independent pharmacies, which purchase smaller volumes of generic drugs.

Estimating the Amount Retained by Wholesalers and Discounts to Pharmacies

The AMP incorporates all discounts given to pharmacies. For generic drugs, therefore, the difference between the average price paid by independent pharmacies and the AMP represents both the wholesalers' markup as well as the average of any off-invoice discounts given to pharmacies for stocking their drugs.[39] In its comparison, CBO used average prices paid by independent pharmacies, rather than the transfer prices reported by chain warehouses, because they are closer to representing actual market-based prices. In percentage terms, the difference between the AMP and the average price paid by independent pharmacies was greatest for generic drugs (see Table 5). On average, for generic drugs, the AMP was 68 percent of the average price paid by independent pharmacies (weighted by sales). For 10 percent of the sales to independent pharmacies, that figure was 39 percent or less, and for another 10 percent, it was 92 percent or more. Those extreme values suggest that the amount retained by pharmacies and wholesalers, as reflected by the gap between the average price paid by independent pharmacies and the AMP, varies widely among generic drugs. For multiple-source brand-name drugs, some variation in those values existed. For single-source drugs, for which manufacturers have little incentive to give pharmacies an off-invoice discount, the average was 95 percent, and there was much less variation around that average.

What may be more relevant, however, is the dollar difference between the AMP and the average price paid by independent pharmacies. In dollar terms, the gap between the two prices was almost as large for single-source drugs as it was for other types of drugs, and it varied as much for single-source drugs as for other drug

---

36. See Federal Trade Commission, *Pharmacy Benefit Managers*, p. 36.

37. See, for example, David Reiffen and Michael Ward, "Generic Drug Industry Dynamics," *The Review of Economics and Statistics*, vol. 87, no. 1 (2005), pp. 37–49. If a generic drug becomes available before all of the brand-name drug's patents have expired, there may be a period of limited competition. Occasionally, a manufacturer of a brand-name drug authorizes a generic version to be sold during that period as well. For more information on patent challenges and how manufacturers of generic drugs can enter the market before all patents have expired, see Federal Trade Commission, *Generic Drug Entry Prior to Patent Expiration* (July 2002).

38. See also Federal Trade Commission, *Pharmacy Benefit Managers*, p. 46. An exception occurs for generic drugs purchased by a PBM for its mail-order pharmacy, in which case the PBM may receive discounts off of the invoice prices.

39. Under current regulations issued by CMS, all discounts to pharmacies are included in the AMP. However, CMS is going to revisit the definition of the AMP, as required by the Deficit Reduction Act of 2005.

Table 5.

The Average Manufacturer Price as a Percentage of the Average Price Paid by Independent Pharmacies

(Percentage of independent pharmacies' price)

Drug Type	Average	Median	By Percentile of Sales			
			10th	25th	75th	90th
Single-Source Brand-Name Drugs	95	97	90	95	98	98
Multiple-Source Brand-Name Drugs	88	94	73	91	97	98
Generic Drugs	68	67	39	56	79	92

Source: Congressional Budget Office based on data from IMS Health for the fourth quarter of 2003.

Notes: Estimates weighted by sales to independent pharmacies.

The average manufacturer price is the price that manufacturers receive on sales to conventional and mail-order pharmacies, including all discounts given to pharmacies and wholesalers.

The price paid by independent pharmacies is the average price they paid to wholesalers, including wholesalers' markups. The pharmacies may receive discounts or rebates from wholesalers or manufacturers that are not included.

types. Because single-source drugs are much more expensive than other types of drugs, a small change in percentage terms between the AMP and the average price paid by independent pharmacies has a large effect on the dollar gap. On a per-prescription basis, the gap averaged $3.80 for single-source brand-name drugs, $4.50 for multiple-source brand-name drugs, $5.00 for new generic drugs, and $1.40 for older generic drugs.[40] And there was considerable variation around those averages among all drug types. Given the structure of incentives in the markets, wholesalers probably obtain most of the difference for single-source drugs, while pharmacies are more likely to obtain a share of that difference for multiple-source drugs, for which they have more influence on what is actually dispensed.[41]

List Prices as Predictors of Transaction Prices

A second distinction of the generic drug market is that the list prices of drugs (such as the AWP and the WAC) are not good predictors of pharmacies' acquisition costs. Payments to pharmacies for generic drugs are based on

list prices. Manufacturers of those drugs may compete for pharmacies' business not only on acquisition costs but also on the gap between acquisition costs and payment rates. Manufacturers may publish relatively high list prices with an eye toward maintaining high payment rates for pharmacies relative to the actual acquisition costs. The result is that transaction prices like the AMP and the average price paid by independent pharmacies are relatively low when compared with the AWP. In CBO's analysis, the AMP was just 25 percent of the AWP for generic drugs, as a sales-weighted average (see Table 6). Considerable variation around that average existed, making predicting actual transaction prices on the basis of list prices difficult.

For single-source brand-name drugs, the sales-weighted average was 79 percent, with much less variation around that average. For brand-name drugs generally, list prices are a more reliable way of setting payment rates to pharmacies than they are for generic drugs. However, even for single-source drugs, a small change in percentage terms can still translate into a relatively large change in the dollar amount that pharmacies and wholesalers retain per prescription. Manufacturers of multiple-source brand-name drugs may also have an incentive to maintain higher list prices relative to transaction prices once their drugs face competition from generic versions. Consistent with that hypothesis, for a share of multiple-source brand-name drugs, the AMP as a percentage of the AWP was low, at 32 percent or less for 10 percent of the sales through independent pharmacies.

---

40. Those reported averages are weighted by the estimated number of prescriptions, obtained for each drug by dividing the number of tablets or capsules sold by the average size of a prescription based on Medicaid data. For multiple-source drugs, the estimates include a small number of instances in which the estimated average price paid by independent pharmacies was less than the reported AMP.

41. An exception might be chain pharmacies, which internalize the wholesale function and thus obtain part of that difference in price for both single-source and multiple-source drugs.

Table 6.

The Average Manufacturer Price and the Average Price Paid by Independent Pharmacies as a Percentage of the Average Wholesale Price

(Percentage of AWP)

	Average	Median	By Percentile of Sales			
			10th	25th	75th	90th
Single-Source Brand-Name Drugs						
Average manufacturer price	79	80	73	78	81	82
Independent pharmacies' price	82	83	80	82	83	84
Multiple-Source Brand-Name Drugs						
Average manufacturer price	69	78	32	69	81	82
Independent pharmacies' price	82	84	80	81	85	86
Generic Drugs						
Average manufacturer price	25	24	4	9	41	48
Independent pharmacies' price	41	48	8	19	61	67

Source: Congressional Budget Office based on data from IMS Health for the fourth quarter of 2003.

Notes: AWP = average wholesale price.

The comparison between the average manufacturer price and the AWP was weighted by sales to all retail pharmacies; the comparison between the average price paid by independent pharmacies and the AWP was weighted by sales to independent pharmacies.

The average manufacturer price is the price that manufacturers receive on sales to conventional and mail-order pharmacies, including all discounts given to pharmacies and wholesalers.

The price paid by independent pharmacies is the average price they paid to wholesalers, including wholesalers' markups. The pharmacies may receive discounts or rebates from wholesalers or manufacturers that are not included.

Overall, then, list prices are not good predictors of actual transaction prices for generic drugs, as they are for single-source brand-name drugs. Hence, it is more difficult for third-party payers to set reimbursement rates based on pharmacies' actual acquisition costs for generic drugs.

PBMs' Payments to Pharmacies

PBMs working on behalf of health plans attempt to account for the artificially high list prices of multiple-source drugs in setting their payment rates to pharmacies for those drugs. PBMs usually set a single maximum allowable cost (MAC) that is the basis for their payments to pharmacies for the ingredient costs of all generic versions of the same drug (with the same active ingredient, dosage form, and strength). PBMs' payments to pharmacies will be equal to the MAC plus a dispensing fee. The MAC is informed by all of the list prices of the different generic versions of the same drug and may also take into consideration other pricing data that PBMs may have on pharmacies' acquisition costs. So whereas the PBMs' payment to pharmacies for a single-source brand-name drug will depend upon the drug's list price, the payment for a generic drug and its brand-name counterpart may depend on a MAC, which is based on one of the lowest list prices among competing generic products.

With respect to multiple-source brand-name drugs, PBMs usually try to minimize their use because generic copies are available. PBMs usually do not negotiate for rebates on such drugs but instead encourage pharmacies to dispense the generic versions.[42] Because the MAC typically applies, dispensing the brand-name drugs is usually unprofitable. However, if a physician writes a prescription specifying "brand only" or "dispense as written," then the pharmacy must either dispense the brand-name product or contact the physician to obtain permission to dispense a generic version. In cases when the pharmacy must dispense the multiple-source brand-name drug, the PBM will usually reimburse the pharmacy on the basis of the AWP for the brand-name drug plus a dispensing fee. And the beneficiary may not have to pay the difference between the cost of the brand-name drug and its generic counterpart.

---

42. Federal Trade Commission, *Pharmacy Benefit Managers*, p. 54.

Appendix:
Data and Methodology Used in This Analysis

Data

The Congressional Budget Office (CBO) estimated the average price paid by different purchasers in the fourth quarter of 2003 for a sample of single-source prescription drugs in oral solid dosage forms (that is, tablets and capsules) relative to their list prices. The sample included more than 170 such drugs defined by their active ingredients—a group that accounted for about 40 percent of all U.S. drug sales in 2003. The analysis also examined the pricing of about 200 multiple-source drugs, which accounted for an additional 7 percent of sales in 2003. Thus, the combined sample covered almost half of drug sales in 2003.

The analysis drew upon data from several different sources. The data came from two private companies that collect and sell information about the pharmaceutical industry, IMS Health and Thomson Micromedex, and from the Centers for Medicare & Medicaid Services (CMS).

IMS Health's National Sales Perspectives

CBO purchased IMS Health's National Sales Perspectives data set for 90 therapeutic classes that included a majority of the top 200 outpatient drugs sold in 2003 and their closely related therapeutic substitutes.[1] The data set was designed to cover most top-selling drugs in oral solid dosage forms and their close therapeutic substitutes. Data included dollar sales at wholesale prices and extended units of drugs (by national drug code, or NDC) purchased in the United States by both retail pharmacies and nonretail providers, by quarter, for 1999 through 2003.[2] The 90 therapeutic classes accounted for about 60 percent of U.S. sales at wholesale prices.

---

1. The data set included 76 of the top 100 outpatient drugs and 117 of the top 200.

Thomson Micromedex's *Red Book*

CBO subscribes to Thomson Micromedex's *Red Book* database. The database contains the average wholesale price (AWP) and the wholesale acquisition cost (WAC) for prescription and nonprescription drugs, by NDC, with dates for when the price went into effect, as well as other prices and descriptive information.

Medicaid's Drug Rebate Program Data

CMS provided CBO with quarterly data for the Medicaid drug rebate program. The data included the average manufacturer price (AMP) and the best price for drugs covered by Medicaid, by NDC. The AMP and the best price are private-sector transaction prices reported by manufacturers to CMS so that it can calculate the Medicaid rebate. The AMP in each quarter is the average price paid to manufacturers by wholesalers (or by pharmacies that buy directly from manufacturers) during that period for drugs distributed to retail and mail-order pharmacies. The best price in each quarter is the lowest price paid to the manufacturers by any private-sector purchaser (excluding Medicare Part D plans). The AMP and the best price are not publicly available data.[3] The information from CMS included data on the prescriptions for and units dispensed to Medicaid recipients and payments to pharmacies by state Medicaid programs.

---

2. Retail pharmacies include independent pharmacies, chain pharmacies, food stores with pharmacies, and mail-order pharmacies. Nonretail providers include nonfederal hospitals, federal facilities, clinics, health maintenance organizations, home health care providers, nursing homes, prisons, universities, and other providers not covered elsewhere.

3. The Deficit Reduction Act of 2005 requires that CMS make AMPs publicly available.

Methodology

To determine the weighted average price relative to the AWP for single-source drugs, CBO calculated the ratio of the cost of buying the quantities of the drugs in the sample at each price—the WAC, the AMP, the best price, and the average prices paid by the different types of retail pharmacies (chain pharmacies, independent pharmacies, food stores with pharmacies, and mail-order pharmacies) and nonretail providers (hospitals, health maintenance organizations, clinics, home health care providers, nursing homes, and federal facilities)—divided by the cost of buying them at the AWP. The mathematical expression for this calculation is

$$\text{Weighted Average Price}_k \text{ Relative to AWP} =$$

$$\frac{\sum (P_{k,i}) \bullet (Q_i)}{\sum (AWP_i) \bullet (Q_i)}$$

where the subscript k represents one of the prices under study (WAC, AMP, best price, and average prices paid by the different retail pharmacies and nonretail providers), where Σ denotes the sum over all drugs in the sample, P is the price per drug, Q is the U.S. quantity of the drug product (for example, the number of tablets or capsules), and the subscript i represents the drug (defined by its trade name, strength, and dosage form—for example, Lipitor 10 mg tablet).

Estimating Prices for Drugs

Some of the prices studied are published (or appear on a publicly available list) and are in effect for a specified period of time. Those include the AWP and the WAC. CBO chose the AWP and the WAC in effect at the midpoint of the fourth quarter of 2003 to represent the AWP and the WAC for that quarter.[4] Thomson Micromedex's *Red Book* lists AWPs and WACs, by NDC, with a date that indicates when they went into effect. The AMPs and the best prices are quarterly prices based on sales to private-sector purchasers over a given quarter.

For each quarter, CBO averaged the AWP, the WAC, the AMP, and the best price across drug package sizes, weighting by the number of tablets or capsules sold in the

---

4.   For this analysis, November 15, 2003, was the midpoint of the fourth quarter.

United States for each package size. That calculation created an average price ($P_{k,i}$) for each brand-name drug at the strength and dosage form for each of the prices—AWP, WAC, AMP, and best price.

The IMS data included dollar and unit sales data from manufacturers, wholesalers, and chain warehouses for each of the different types of retail pharmacies and nonretail providers. For each of the different types of retail pharmacies and nonretail providers and for each drug product, CBO summed expenditures for all package sizes and divided by the total number of tablets or capsules summed for all package sizes to create average prices for each drug for each of the different types of retail pharmacies and nonretail providers ($P_{k,i}$).

Weighting by U.S. Quantities

The average prices (AWP, WAC, AMP, best price, and average prices paid by the different retail pharmacies and nonretail providers) were matched with data on the total units sold in the United States (Q_i) for each product. Drugs with any one of the average prices missing were deleted, resulting in a final data set with 456 drug products when defined by trade name, strength, and dosage form (for example, Lipitor 10 mg tablet), or 178 drugs when defined by trade name alone. Following the formula for a price index, CBO estimated weighted-average prices relative to the AWP, using the number of tablets or capsules sold in the United States of each product as the weight.

Analysis of the Pricing of Multiple-Source Drugs

The methodological approach for analyzing the pricing of multiple-source drugs differed from that used for single-source drugs. For multiple-source drugs, CBO computed sales-weighted averages and distributions of specific price ratios (presented in percentage terms in Tables 5 and 6). CBO chose that alternative approach to capture the greater variance in pricing relationships among multiple-source drugs compared with those among single-source drugs.

For example, dollar sales to independent pharmacies were used to weight the ratio of the AMP to the price paid by independent pharmacies). The formula for estimating a sales-weighted average is

$$\frac{\sum (AMP_i / INDEP_i) \bullet S_i}{\sum S_i}$$

where AMP_i is the average manufacturer price of drug (i), $INDEP_i$ is the price paid by independent pharmacies for drug (i), and S_i is the dollar sales to independent pharmacies of drug (i). The sales-weighted median is the value of $AMP_i/INDEP_i$ at the point at which, after the drugs are in rank order by the value of $AMP_i/INDEP_i$, the sum of independent sales up to drug (i) over total sales is equal to 0.5. Similarly, the value of $AMP_i/INDEP_i$ at the 10th percentile is taken at the point at which, after the drugs are in rank order by the value of $AMP_i/INDEP_i$, the sum of independent sales up to drug (i) over total sales is equal to 0.1. Thus, for 10 percent of the sales, the ratio of AMP_i to $INDEP_i$ is less than or equal to the value of $AMP_i/INDEP_i$ at the 10th percentile.

Glossary

Average Manufacturer Price (AMP): The AMP is the average price paid to manufacturers for drugs distributed through retail pharmacies. It includes all forms of discounts given to wholesalers and to pharmacies, but it does not include rebates paid by manufacturers to third-party payers. The AMP is used to calculate the rebates that manufacturers of brand-name drugs are required to give to federal and state governments for sales to Medicaid beneficiaries.

Average Wholesale Price (AWP): A publicly available list price for sales of drugs by wholesalers to pharmacies or other providers, the AWP is not the actual price that wholesalers charge but is more like a sticker price in the automobile industry. The AWP is used as the basis for setting payment rates to pharmacies. This study relied on the AWPs published in Thomson Micromedex's *Red Book*.

Best Price: The best price is used to calculate the rebates that manufacturers of brand-name drugs are required to pay to state Medicaid programs on sales to Medicaid beneficiaries. The best price is the lowest price paid by any private-sector purchaser (excluding Medicare prescription drug plans), and it includes discounts, rebates, and other pricing adjustments.

Brand-Name Drug: In this study, a brand-name drug is usually one that has received a patent on its chemical entity, formulation, or use; has been approved by the Food and Drug Administration after clinical testing; and is sold under a brand name. It is a single-source drug while it is still protected by its patent and becomes a multiple-source drug once generic versions become available.

Charge-Back: Manufacturers negotiate discounted prices with some purchasers who buy through wholesalers. Wholesalers can deliver the drugs at discounted prices, inform the manufacturers, and then request reimbursement from the manufacturers. Such discounts handled through wholesalers are generally known as charge-backs.

Conventional Pharmacy: For the purposes of this study, conventional pharmacies include chain pharmacies, independent pharmacies, and pharmacies in food stores but exclude mail-order pharmacies.

Discounts: A mechanism, such as a charge-back or prompt-pay discount, that lowers the net price of a drug at the time of purchase.

Formulary: A formulary is a list of drugs approved for coverage under a drug benefit. Pharmacy benefit managers (PBMs) working on behalf of health plans determine which drugs are therapeutically similar. Then, for such brand-name drugs with several close substitutes, PBMs negotiate with manufacturers for lower prices and rebates in return for placing the manufacturers' drugs on their formularies.

The patients served by a PBM may have access to only those drugs on a formulary (in the case of a closed formulary) or may have access to all prescription drugs but at different levels of copayments or other conditions (in the case of an open formulary).

Each of those functions may also be undertaken by the health plan itself, rather than by a PBM. Some nonretail providers, such as hospitals, also use formularies.

Generic Drug: A copy of a brand-name drug, containing the same active ingredients that the Food and Drug Administration judges to be comparable in terms of therapeutic effectiveness. Generic copies may be sold after the patent on a brand-name drug has expired. Generic drugs are usually sold under their chemical name rather than under a brand name.

List Price: A list price is a published price that is not an actual transaction price. However certain pharmaceutical transactions, such as setting payment rates to pharmacies, may be based on list prices. The average wholesale price and the wholesale acquisition cost are examples of list prices.

Mail-Order Pharmacy: At the retail level, a mail-order pharmacy dispenses and delivers prescriptions through the mail. Many mail-order pharmacies are owned by pharmacy benefit managers.

Maximum Allowable Cost (MAC): A MAC is an upper payment limit on the ingredient costs for a multiple-source drug. PBMs set MACs for the purpose of reimbursing pharmacies. All generic drugs with the same active ingredients, strength, and dosage form will have the same MAC.

Multiple-Source Drug: A multiple-source drug is one available in both brand-name and generic versions from a variety of manufacturers.

Nonretail Provider: In this study, nonretail providers include hospitals, health maintenance organizations (HMOs), clinics, home health care providers, nursing homes, and federal facilities.

Pharmacy Benefit Manager (PBM): PBMs administer drug benefits on behalf of health plans and employers. They negotiate with both pharmacies and manufacturers for lower prices. By adopting formularies, PBMs obtain discounted prices on many brand-name drugs in the form of rebates from manufacturers, which are shared with health plans.

Rebate Payment: Manufacturers may provide to nonretail providers, pharmacies, PBMs, health plans, or any third-party payers rebate payments that reduce the net prices of drugs. Those payments occur after the purchases of the drugs and are usually confidential.

Single-Source Drug: A single-source drug is under patent protection and sold under a brand name—and thus is available from only one manufacturer (or occasionally from other manufacturers under license from the patent holder). No generic version is available.

Third-Party Payer: In the case of health insurance coverage, a third-party payer is the source of payment for health benefits. For drug coverage, the third-party payer is usually a health plan, health maintenance organization, self-insured employer, or a government program such as Medicaid.

Wholesale Acquisition Cost (WAC): A publicly available list price for sales of drugs by manufacturers to wholesalers. The WAC is not, as its name suggests, what wholesalers pay for drugs; instead, it approximates what retail pharmacies pay wholesalers for single-source drugs. This study relied on the WAC for drugs published in Thomson Micromedex's *Red Book*.